SKILLS UPDATE

BARBARA STILWELL

Illustrated by Mike Bostock

Edited by
Sue Smith, Editor
Community Outlook

Designed by
Hilary Tranter

First edition 1992
Reprinted 1992
Reprinted 1993
Reprinted 1995
Reprinted 1996

Published by
Macmillan Magazines Ltd
Porters South
Crinan Street
London N1 9XW

Printed in Great Britain by Pro Litho, London

ISBN 0-333-57861-9

CONTENTS

MEASURING BLOOD PRESSURE

PHYSIOLOGY OF BLOOD PRESSURE

There are several physiological components which affect blood pressure:

■ The heart. With each beat, blood is pumped from the left ventricle to the aorta. This raises the blood pressure to its *systolic* pressure. When the heart is relaxed, it is said to be in diastole and the *diastolic* pressure is heard
■ The aorta and other large arteries dilate to accommodate each pulse of blood. If the arteries are narrowed or rigid, systolic pressure will be raised (for example, in arteriosclerosis)
■ The peripheral arteries carry the blood from the aorta to the arterioles and the capillaries. The smooth muscle around these vessels can contract to raise blood pressure by narrowing the blood vessel

■ The kidney produces renin, an enzyme, which in turn converts angiotensin to an active vasopressor substance. This causes constriction of the blood vessels and affects the retention of salt and fluid by the kidney, increasing the total blood volume and thus raising blood pressure
■ The sympathetic nervous system exerts control over blood pressure through alpha- and beta-receptors

If you are unclear about the physiology of blood pressure, it will help you to read about it in full again. See also 'Systems of Life' series in *Nursing Times* 1990; **86**: 46, 24–28, and *Nursing Times* 1990; **86**: 50, 53–56.

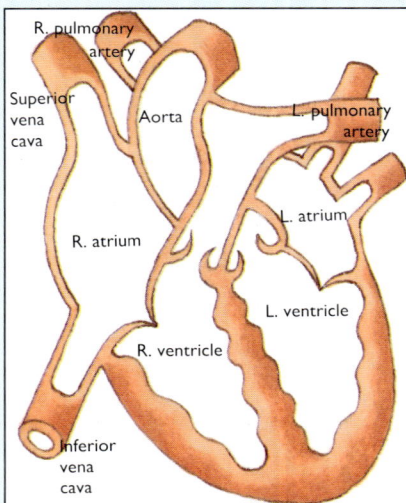

Anatomy of the heart

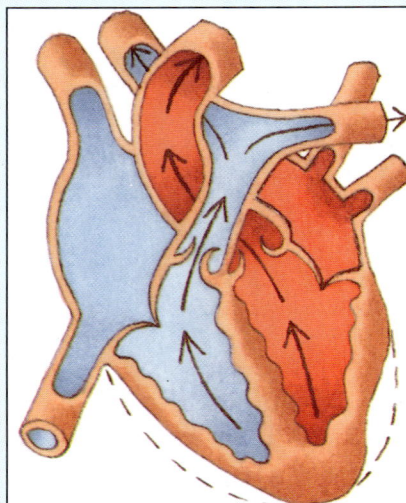

R. pulmonary artery
Superior vena cava
Aorta
L. pulmonary artery
R. atrium
L. atrium
L. ventricle
R. ventricle
Inferior vena cava

Ventricular systole

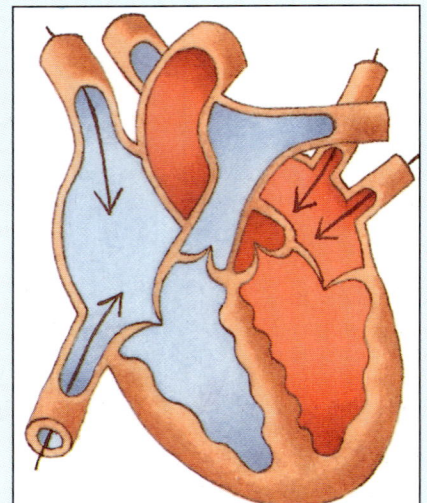

Diastole — the resting heart

TAKING BLOOD PRESSURE

Because decisions about treatment are based on small differences in blood pressure, it is important that it is measured consistently and accurately.

- Ideally the patient should be allowed to sit down for 15 minutes before blood pressure is measured
- The patient should be sitting comfortably with his arm supported. Blood pressure is higher when the patient is standing
- The sphygmomanometer cuff should be applied at the level of the heart and there should be no tight clothing constricting the arm above it
- The cuff should be large enough. The standard cuff is adequate for an arm of up to 275 mm in circumference. If the cuff is too small, the blood pressure reading will be artificially raised
- The cuff should be inflated above (but only just above) the anticipated level of the systolic pressure. This can be checked by feeling the radial or brachial pulse
- The cuff should be deflated slowly, so that the column of mercury falls at approximately 2 mm per second
- The observer should have her eyes level with the vertical column of mercury to avoid parallax error
- The blood pressure should be recorded to the nearest 2 mmHg
- The systolic blood pressure should be recorded when the sounds are first heard (Korotkoff Phase I) and the diastolic blood pressure when the sounds disappear (Korotkoff Phase V)

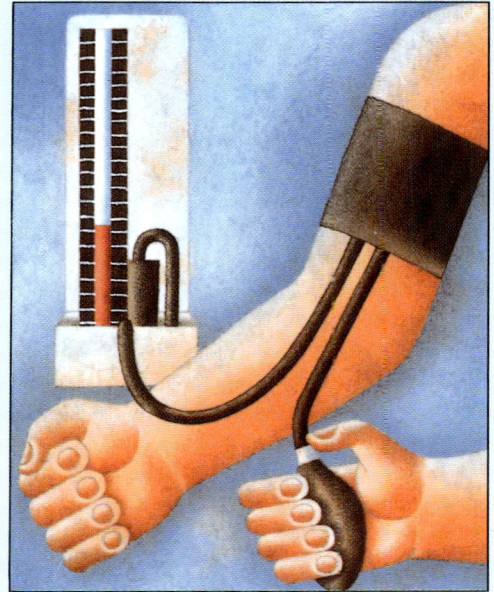

ERRORS IN TAKING BLOOD PRESSURE OCCUR IF:

- The machine is poorly maintained. The column should be cleaned at regular intervals and the mercury should rest at zero. Its accuracy should be checked at regular intervals against other machines
- The column is allowed to drop too quickly or too slowly
- Blood pressure is read only to the nearest 5 or 10 mmHg
- The observer is influenced by previous readings to record a result which is consistent with them
- The patient has a full bladder
- The patient is anxious or angry (blood pressure up), cold (blood pressure up) or hot (blood pressure down)

WHAT LEVEL IS HIGH?

World Health Organisation criteria for hypertension (mmHg)

	Systolic BP	Diastolic BP
Normal	<140	<90
Borderline	140–159	90–94
Definite	>160	>94
Mild hypertension	160–179	95–104

Blood pressure that is above normal limits should be reassessed twice and the mean reading calculated. This is because blood pressure can be influenced by many changing factors. Patients whose diastolic blood pressure is above 105 mmHg on three occasions should be encouraged to take treatment.

OTHER FACTORS THAT AFFECT BLOOD PRESSURE

- Age. The arteries lose their elasticity with increasing age. People who have high blood pressure when young have higher blood pressure when old; therefore people with marginally raised blood pressure should be carefully monitored as they get older
- Heredity. Up to 50% of people with raised blood pressure have an inherited predisposition. It is important to take a family history
- Weight. Increased weight can cause blood pressure to rise. It is important, therefore, to weigh and measure a person with raised blood pressure and check whether they are overweight
- Alcohol intake. A high alcohol intake is linked to high blood pressure
- Anything that compromises the physiology that maintains normal blood pressure

YOU SHOULD NOW FEEL COMPETENT TO:

- Measure blood pressure accurately to the nearest 2 mmHg
- Assess reasons why blood pressure might be high
- Know when to refer for further assessment and treatment

FURTHER READING

1 Sorensen, K., Luckmann, J. Basic Nursing: A Psychophysiologic Approach. Philadelphia, Pa.: W. B. Saunders, 1986.
2 Stilwell, B., Hobbs, R. Nursing in General Practice: Clinical Care. Oxford: Radcliffe Medical Press, 1990.

INJECTIONS

WHO MAY PRESENT?

- People needing drugs administered by a parenteral route (for example, insulin, cyanocobalamin, Depo injections, penicillin)
- People needing tests done by intradermal injection (for example, Schick test, Mantoux test)
- Those needing vaccinations and immunisations, including babies and children.

PARENTERAL ROUTES

Injectable drugs may be given:
- Between the layers of skin — intradermal, for example, for Schick tests
- Into subcutaneous tissue — subcutaneous, for example, for insulin
- Into a muscle — intramuscular, for example, for antibiotics
- Into a vein (not dealt with in this update).

WHEN INJECTING DRUGS

YOU NEED TO KNOW

- Has the drug that is to be injected been prescribed?
- Does the patient have an intolerance to the drug to be injected?
- Does the drug have any rapid side-effects, such as anaphylaxis?
- Are you giving the correct drug?
- Are you administering the drug to be injected by the correct route?

YOU SHOULD THEREFORE

- Check the notes or prescription for drug and dosage
- Ask the patient if the drug has been given before
- Find out whether the patient has any allergies
- Know how to deal with anaphylaxis
- Check the box and ampoule to make sure it is the right drug
- Check the 'use-by' date
- Check the information enclosed with the drug to make sure you are administering by the correct route.

IF YOU ARE IN DOUBT ABOUT ANY OF THIS INFORMATION, CHECK WITH A QUALIFIED NURSING OR MEDICAL COLLEAGUE

NOW YOU SHOULD SELECT A ROUTE TO G

INTRADERMAL INJECTIONS

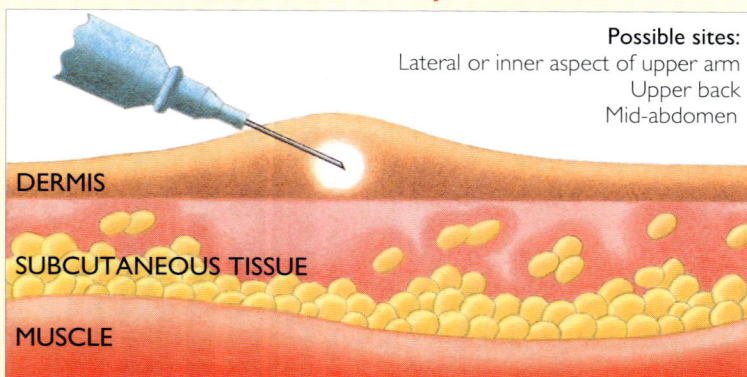

Possible sites:
Lateral or inner aspect of upper arm
Upper back
Mid-abdomen

DERMIS

SUBCUTANEOUS TISSUE

MUSCLE

Criteria for selection:
- As for subcutaneous injection and in addition:
- The site to be injected should be free of excessive pigmentation
- The site to be injected should be relatively hairless.

SUBCUTANEOUS INJECTIONS

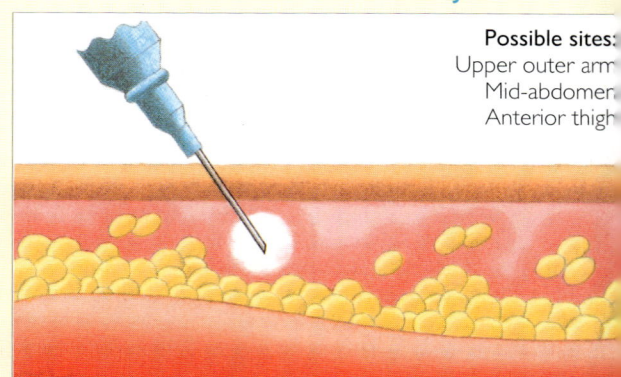

Possible sites:
Upper outer arm
Mid-abdomen
Anterior thigh

Criteria for selection:
- The site should not overlie large muscles, nerves or bon prominences
- Skin should be free of painful or hard lumps from previo injections (rotate sites if frequent injections are required
- The subcutaneous tissue at the site should be thick enou to accommodate the volume of drug.

GIVING THE INJECTION

- Wash your hands, and use sterile equipment.
- Use a suitable sized needle: viscous fluids require a larger-gauge needle; deeper injections require a longer needle.
- Clean the skin if it is dirty and you are not giving an immunisation.
- Visualise where the drug is to go (that is, by what route) and angle the needle accordingly.
- Some drugs given intramuscularly irritate the subcutaneous tissues. Therefore draw up the drug using one needle, then change it to inject.
- Pulling the skin taut before injecting stretches the small nerves under the skin and makes the procedure less painful.
- Letting an anxious patient lie down may avert a vaso-vagal attack.
- Consider using an anaesthetic cream if the patient is very nervous or a child. Time needs to be allowed for the anaesthetic to take effect.

POINTS TO NOTE

- Symptoms of anaphylactic shock include difficulty in breathing, low blood pressure, tachycardia or arrhythmia, oedema of the face, larynx and tongue and itching of the skin. Adrenaline 1:1000 should be given by deep intramuscular injection. This must be available at all times in the treatment room, together with a Brook airway.
- Injections for children are less painful if the child is securely held by a parent. The child's legs should be enclosed by the parent's legs, and his arms 'cuddled' by the parent's arms. He should be told that it will probably hurt for just a moment.
- It is not necessary to massage the injection site after the injection; it serves no useful purpose and may cause pain and bruising.

INJECTION SITES

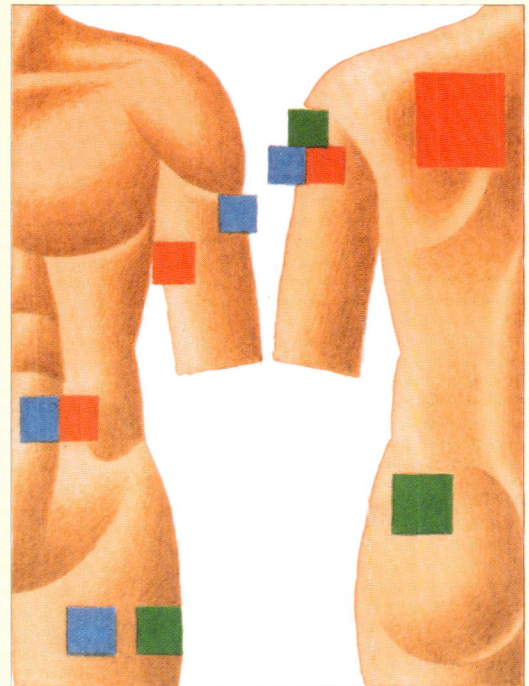

KEY
- Intradermal
- Subcutaneous
- Intramuscular

INJECTION

INTRAMUSCULAR INJECTIONS

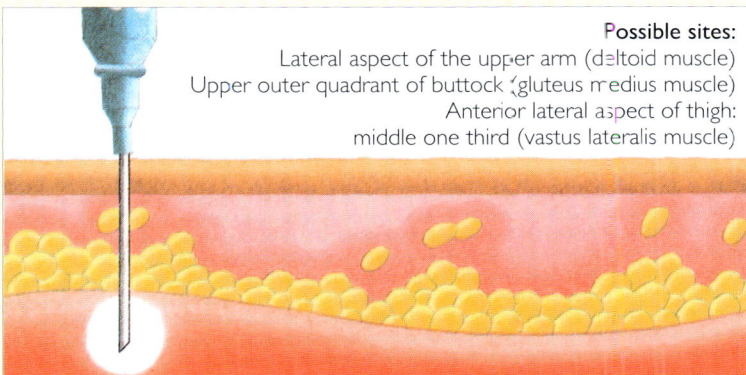

Possible sites:
Lateral aspect of the upper arm (deltoid muscle)
Upper outer quadrant of buttock (gluteus medius muscle)
Anterior lateral aspect of thigh:
middle one third (vastus lateralis muscle)

Criteria for selection:
- The muscle must be large enough to accommodate the volume of solution to be given. A full-grown client with well-developed muscles can tolerate an injected volume of 3 ml without discomfort
- There must be no danger of the needle striking a nerve, bone or major blood vessel
- The selected muscle should be free of tender or hard lesions on palpation
- The client should be in a position that relaxes the muscle.

NOW YOU SHOULD FEEL COMPETENT TO:

- Administer drugs safely by a variety of parenteral routes — intradermally, subcutaneously and intramuscularly.
- Ensure the patient's comfort and safety throughout the procedure of giving the injection, whether the patient is an adult or a child.

FURTHER READING
Department of Health. *Immunisation Against Infectious Diseases.* London: HMSO, 1990.
British Medical Association and Royal Pharmaceutical Society of Great Britain. *British National Formulary.* London: British Medical Association and Royal Pharmaceutical Society of Great Britain, 1992.

NON-INSULIN-DE

WHO MAY PRESENT

- Patients who have been identified as having non-insulin-dependent diabetes (NIDD) who are usually over 40 years of age, overweight and, most often, women.

TESTING BLOOD SUGAR

- Capillary blood can be tested in the clinic, using glucose strips, such as BM Stix. The strip can be read manually or by using a meter. Accurate timing in the use of glucose strips is important. and the blood should fall on to the strip rather than be 'wiped on'. The glycosylated haemaglobin is a reliable indicator of blood sugar control over the preceding three months. Blood for this should be collected in a 5 ml EDTA tube. Lipid levels should also be checked.

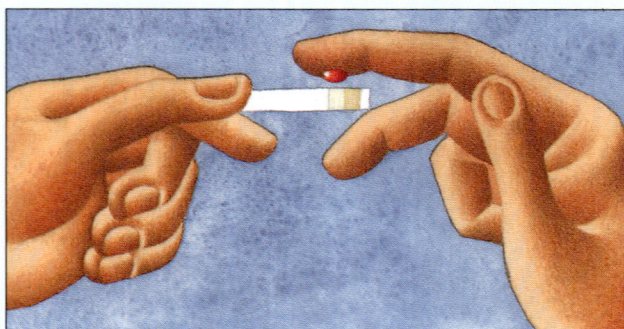

GENERAL CONSIDERATIONS

- The majority of people who have NIDD will be overweight. Control of obesity is an effective way of treating NIDD, and two-thirds of patients could achieve a normal glucose tolerance test after six months of good dietary control.
- In a practice population of 1000, you could expect there to be eight people with diabetes, of whom six would not be insulin dependent.
- Having NIDD increases the risk of developing cardiovascular disease: people with diabetes have higher blood pressures than non-diabetics.
- Some drugs can cause a raised blood sugar. These include beta-blockers, steroids, diuretics and oral contraceptives. If these are the precipitating factor, withdrawal of the drug is required to bring the blood sugar levels under control.
- The presentation of NIDD is usually gradual, with symptoms including a mild thirst, possibly polyuria and nocturia and sometimes pruritis vulvae or recurrent boils. However, there may be no symptoms, which is why it is important to screen the urine of older people for the presence of sugar.
- Diagnosis must be confirmed by a venous blood sugar estimation, rather than capillary blood testing. A random blood sugar level of more than 10 mmol, or a fasting level of more than 6.7 mmol, establishes the diagnosis.
- The majority of people with NIDD can be cared for in general practice either by dietary modification or by oral drug therapy; others with major complications or poor control may need hospital supervision.

SETTING UP A CLINIC

- It is important to stress that this update is not referring to the insulin-dependent diabetic patient.
- It is obviously important to be able to identify those people with NIDD in order to be able to send for them and to follow them up. Many practices now have computers on which these data can be recorded. If not, special records must be kept which show last attendances, next appointments and the type of treatment that the patient is taking.
- The objectives of care in the clinic should be to monitor treatment, prevent complications and to give appropriate education.
- Support should be arranged from a local dietitian. Ideally she should attend the clinic, but if she cannot she should accept referrals. Similarly, a chiropodist should be available for advice and treatment.

Tasks performed at follow-up should include :
- Weighing the client (and recording his or her height measurement if not already done). This is especially important for those people in whom obesity is a predisposing factor in diabetes. Their body mass index (BMI) should be estimated and they should be encouraged to lose weight if necessary until the BMI is 25 or less (see page 17).
- Measuring blood pressure (see page 2).
- Testing the urine for glucose and protein. The presence of protein may be an early sign of secondary damage to the kidneys.
- Recording an electrocardiogram (patients over 40 years).
- Testing visual acuity with a Snellen chart, the patient standing six metres away from the chart. Each eye should be tested separately, looking through a pin-hole if refraction is necessary. There should be annual screening for retinopathy either by the GP, an optician or a hospital screening clinic.
- Inspecting the feet, because one of the complications of diabetes is neuropathy, affecting almost 50% of people with diabetes after 25 years. It can produce a loss of sensation, possibly leading to ulceration and infection. In addition, the feet may become ischaemic, again resulting in ulceration.
- Educating the patient, including information about lifestyle changes which reduce the risk of heart disease and stroke (see page 16). It is especially important for the diabetic patient to stop smoking, and you should offer specific help with this. Patients need to know how to cope with hypo-glycaemia when taking oral hypoglycaemic agents and also that their blood sugar levels may be affected if they are unwell.

DIETARY ADVICE

■ Diet should be as normal as possible. The principles are the same as those of a healthy diet for anyone, and you may be able to persuade a whole family to change its eating habits. The principles are:
— Reduce fat consumption, especially animal fats, and cut surplus fats off meats
— Increase fibre-rich foods, because these tend to slow down the rate of absorption of sugars from the gut. This is most effective with fibre derived from pulses such as beans and lentils
— Ensure that around 50% of calories come from carbohydrates, which should be made up of foods high in roughage such as cereals, pasta and potatoes
— Avoid refined sugars, present in cakes and sweets
— Eat low-fat proteins such as chicken and fish .
■ The overweight person with diabetes will also need to watch calorie intake, restricting it to 1000 calories per day.
■ Ideally all patients should have an initial consultation with a dietitian.

MEASURING PULSE RATES

Taking the dorsalis pedis pulse
■ Feel the dorsum of the foot (not the ankle) just lateral to the exterior tendon of the great toe. If you cannot feel a pulse, explore the dorsum of the foot more laterally.

Taking the posterior tibial pulse
■ Curve your fingers behind and slightly below the medial malleolus of the ankle. (This pulse may be hard to feel in fat or oedematous ankles.)

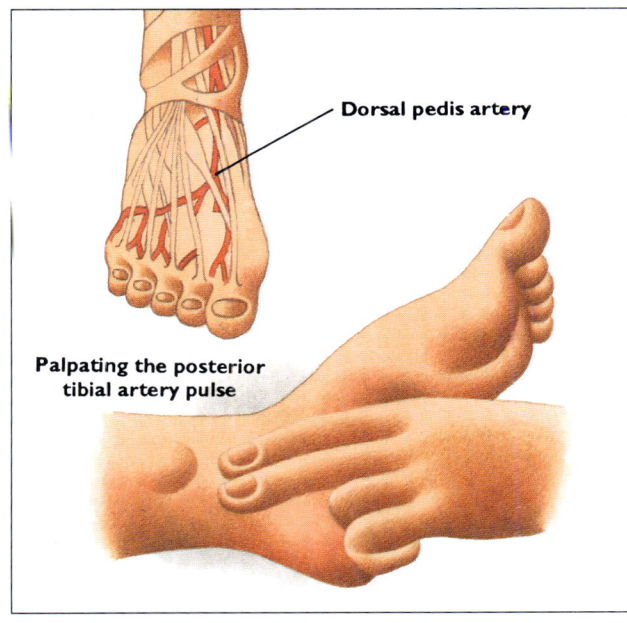

Dorsal pedis artery

Palpating the posterior tibial artery pulse

HOW TO EXAMINE THE FEET

During a foot inspection the nurse should look for:
■ Unnoticed trauma from ill-fitting shoes
■ Burns from hot-water bottles
■ Ulcers caused by pressure, especially on the sole of the feet
■ Claw toes caused by muscle wasting
■ Pink feet and hairless legs (a sign of ischaemia)
■ Thick and hard skin or corns and callouses requiring chiropody
■ Any oedema.

During palpation you should:
■ Feel for the dorsalis pedis pulse and the posterior tibial pulse (see diagram). Decreased or absent pulses suggest occlusion of the arteries and you should refer the patient to a doctor
■ Use the back of your fingers and feel the temperature of the feet. Unilateral coldness particularly suggests arterial insufficiency.

FOOT CARE FOR THE PATIENT

Remind patients to:
■ Examine their feet daily
■ Wash their feet every day with warm, not hot, water and dry carefully between the toes
■ Use a moisturising cream to prevent hard skin
■ Never walk barefoot
■ Wrap up hot-water bottles in a thick towel. Do not put feet near the fire
■ Check shoes each day for stones or hard edges that may go unnoticed
■ Wear well-fitting, broad shoes
■ Consult a chiropodist regularly
■ Cover all cuts or blisters with a sterile non-adhesive dressing.

YOU SHOULD NOW FEEL COMPETENT TO

■ Assess the person with NIDD who is being treated by diet or oral drugs.

Remember that it is important to discuss what you are doing in the clinic with colleagues and to construct a protocol of care. If in any doubt about your assessment, consult a more experienced colleague or a medical practitioner.

Further information is available from the British Diabetic Association, 10 Queen Anne Street, London W1M 0BD.

FURTHER READING
Stilwell, B., Hobbs, R. Nursing in General Practice: Clinical Care, Book 1. Oxford: Radcliffe Medical Press, 1990

TAKING SWABS

WHO MAY PRESENT?

Someone with an infection where the presence of a pathogenic organism is suspected and a differential diagnosis would be helpful in prescribing appropriate treatment.

GENERAL CONSIDERATIONS

■ Swabs are collected so that the microbiologist can identify the pathogen causing an infection. Care must therefore be taken to ensure that the swab is not contaminated by surrounding normal flora.

■ You also need to ensure that you are not contaminated by the swab. You should wear seamless latex gloves and, if taking a swab from the mouth of a patient who is coughing, stand to one side or wear a mask.

■ Swabs can be taken from a range of sites, including the mouth, nasopharynx, wound sites and vagina, and many different organisms can be identified by this method. It is vital that you are familiar with the requirements of your local laboratory for type of swab used, transport medium required, time of collection of swab and whether immediate delivery to the laboratory is necessary. If in doubt, ask.

■ Whenever possible, collect the specimen before antibiotics have been taken. Always note on the form if the patient has had a course of antibiotics and what they were.

HANDLING SPECIMENS

■ All swab containers should be labelled in advance.

■ Take care not to contaminate the outside of the container by touching it with the swab or with a 'dirty' gloved hand.

■ A swab should reach the laboratory as soon as possible after collection while it is still moist. If a delay is unavoidable, the specimen should be placed in a sterile moistening broth to preserve its viability.

■ Some laboratories prefer all the swabs to be transported in a culture medium, and these will be supplied. The type of swabs and transport containers supplied will vary from place to place, depending, often, on the funding of the laboratory. If you are unsure about what you should be using, contact the laboratory and ask for advice or request a procedure manual.

■ Ensure that the form is completed accurately. As well as all the patient's details, it should show the site from where the swab was taken. If it is a wound swab, the nature of the wound should be described (for example, post-operative, animal or human bite, ulcer).

■ If a particular condition is suspected because of the clinical condition of the patient, the form should state this so that the laboratory can look for particular organisms. Remember to note any antibiotics taken.

TAKING A THROAT SWAB

■ The procedure should be quick — to minimise discomfort. You will probably be taking the swab of exudate on the tonsils, so be sure that you are familiar with the anatomy of the mouth and throat.

■ Explain to the patient the reason for this procedure and what it involves. Some people find the sensation of having their throat touched unpleasant, and most people gag during the procedure. Explain that this may be the case and reassure them that this is a normal response.

■ Gather together the equipment you will require. In addition to the swab, you will need a flexible light, gloves and a tongue depressor.

■ Seat the patient so that he or she is comfortable and so that the light gives the best illumination possible.

■ Put on the gloves and loosen the swab from its container. Do not remove it completely — it must remain sterile until the specimen is collected.

■ Obtain a good view of the throat and collect the specimen by gently but firmly rotating the swab in the exudate. The more exudate that there is, the easier the job of the microbiologist.

■ When collecting the specimen, do not touch the lips, cheeks or tongue. Normal flora may contaminate the specimen if you do so.

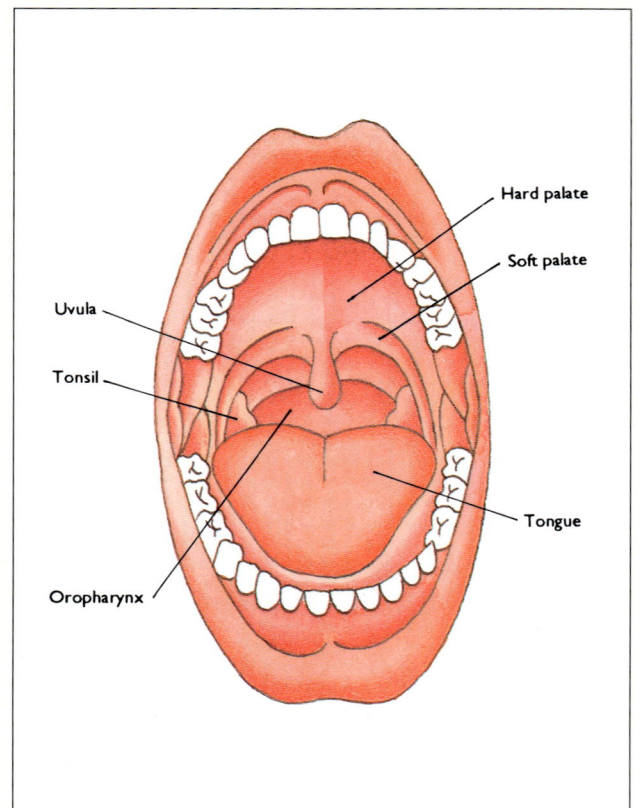

NASOPHARYNGEAL SWABS

■ Nasopharyngeal swabs are sometimes recommended for recovering *Neisseria meningitidis* (meningococcus) or *Bordetella pertussis* (causative agent of whooping cough). These organisms require special culture and this must be specified on the laboratory request form.

■ Nasopharyngeal swabs are long and flexible so that they can be inserted into the nasopharynx via the nose or mouth.

■ Explain the procedure clearly to the patient. If the patient is a child, explain to the parent the necessity for the child to be held as still as possible and show how this can be done.

■ With the patient seated, tilt the head back and use a small torch to obtain a good view of the nasal passages.

■ If the nostrils are narrow, you may have to push the tip of the nose upwards to get a clear view. Alternatively you may need to use a nasal speculum to dilate one nostril. If so, insert the speculum into the nose until the point where the blades begin to widen, then open it gently. Nasal specula should not be used on children.

■ Wearing gloves, insert the swab carefully through the nostril into the nasopharynx and rotate it gently.

■ Withdraw the swab, trying not to contaminate it with other nasal secretions.

■ The swab should be placed in a transport medium and sent immediately to the laboratory.

■ Nasopharyngeal swabs can also be obtained via the mouth. The area which should be swabbed lies below the uvula. It is important not to contaminate the swab when inserting or withdrawing it on the tongue or buccal mucosa.

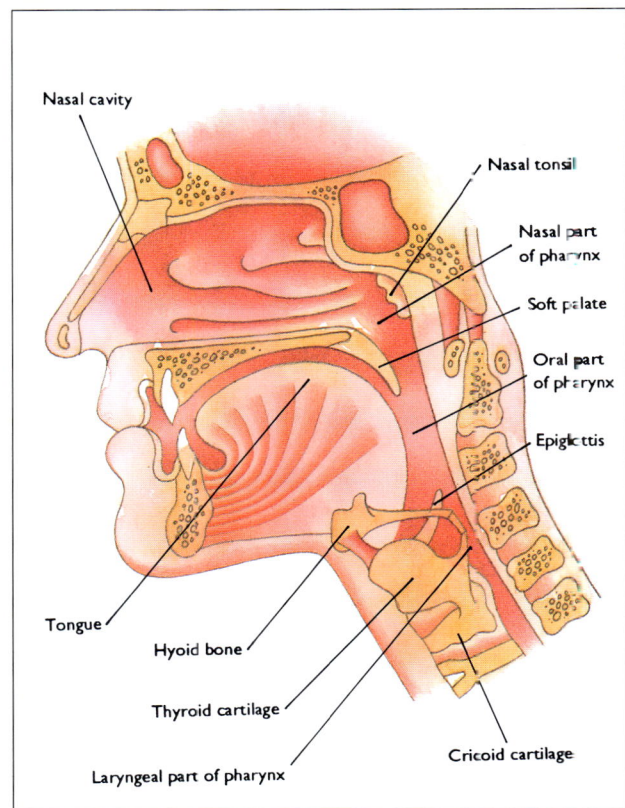

Labels: Nasal cavity, Nasal tonsil, Nasal part of pharynx, Soft palate, Oral part of pharynx, Epiglottis, Tongue, Hyoid bone, Thyroid cartilage, Cricoid cartilage, Laryngeal part of pharynx

TAKING SWABS FROM WOUNDS

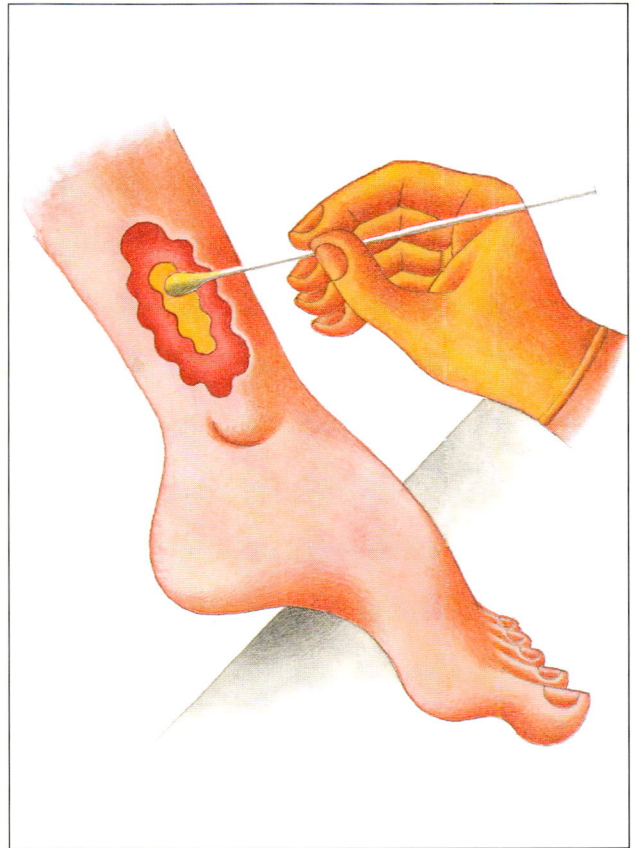

■ If you suspect that a wound is infected because it is inflamed, hot, painful or there is pus present it is advisable to swab the infected area to identify the cause of the infection and establish the antibiotics to which the organism is sensitive.

■ Explain to the patient why you think this procedure is necessary and what it will involve.

■ Expose the wound. Remember to use an aseptic technique to avoid contaminating the swab or yourself.

■ Swab the exudate of the wound, taking care not to touch the surrounding skin

YOU SHOULD NOW FEEL COMPETENT TO:

Take an uncontaminated throat, nasopharyngeal or wound swab suitable for microbiological culture.

FURTHER READING
Kee, J.L. *Laboratory and Diagnostic Tests with Nursing Implications*. Norwalk, Conn,: Appleton-Century-Crofts, 1983.
McGhee, M.F. *A Guide to Laboratory Investigations*. Oxford: Radcliffe Medical Press, 1989.

TREATING ASTHMA

WHO MAY PRESENT?

- An adult or a child who has been diagnosed as having asthma.
- An adult or a child who needs to learn to use inhaled medication.

GENERAL CONSIDERATIONS

- This update deals with lung function tests and the use of inhalers. It is not a substitute for a detailed course in the diagnosis and treatment of asthma, which is essential for nurses who wish to extend their role in the care of asthmatic patients.
- It is worth revising the anatomy and physiology of lung function if you are unclear about either.
- Peak expiratory flow meters are now available on prescription, and one aspect of the nurse's role is to teach people how to measure and record their peak expiratory flow rate at home. It is therefore important to understand this technique fully enough to be able to explain it in simple language.
- It is especially helpful to people with asthma to understand what the disorder is and how the treatment works. In this way, they are more likely to use their inhaled medication as instructed and avoid acute asthma attacks, which should not occur when the disease is well controlled. One important role of the nurse is to explain to patients about their treatment and when they should seek medical advice. Do not underestimate the importance of education for the person with asthma.
- There are many leaflets available to give information to people with asthma. Some of these come from drug companies, but many are non-promotional; write to the makers of drugs used in the treatment of asthma for examples. Write, too, to the National Asthma Campaign and to the British Lung Foundation for examples of their educational material.

WHAT IS ASTHMA?

- Asthma is a reversible airways obstruction.
- In asthma the airways are constricted because bronchial and bronchiolar smooth muscle contract and narrow the lumen in the bronchi and bronchioles.
- There may be oversecretion of mucous in the airways, resulting in further obstruction.
- In addition, the lining of the bronchi and bronchioles may become swollen and inflamed and the airways further narrowed.
- Asthma may be provoked by an allergy, by chemical triggers such as smoke or workplace environment, by infection or through exertion.
- The symptoms of asthma include wheezing, shortness of breath and coughing. Not all of these may be present, and it is most important that peak flow rate is measured accurately because the diagnosis of asthma may be confirmed by this measurement of airflow obstruction.

MEASURING PEAK EXPIRATORY FLOW RATE

- The peak flow rate is the maximum rate of expiration occurring within the first second of forced expiration, so the patient will be required to exhale quickly and with force.
- Peak flow rate is dependent on age, sex, height, build and posture. Accurate measurement depends on good technique.
- Explain to the patient what the test involves and why it is being done.
- The patient should be standing in order to allow the diaphragm to move freely and the lungs to expand fully.
- Check that the pointer is on zero.
- Instruct the patient to hold the meter horizontally and not to put his or her fingers over the pointer.
- The patient should take a deep breath in and put the mouthpiece between the lips, which must be tightly sealed around it.
- The patient should blow suddenly and hard.
- Read the position of the pointer and then repeat the test twice more, noting the best of the three readings.
- If the patient is a child, demonstration is vital, as is enlisting the help of the parent in winning trust and cooperation. Getting children to blow out candles is a very good way of demonstrating the need for a short, sharp exhalation. Paediatric peak flow meters are available and have small mouthpieces.

INHALED DRUGS

- Delivery systems which allow a drug to be inhaled are widely used in the treatment of asthma. This is because an inhaled drug is transported to the bronchi immediately, where it works more quickly and has fewer side-effects.
- There are several devices available to deliver inhaled drugs; these include aerosols (metered dose inhalers), breath-activated devices such as Autohaler, and devices which deliver dry powder such as Spinhaler. Spacers, such as Volumatic and Nebuhaler, are used with an aerosol; the spray from the aerosol is released into a plastic chamber, so the patient breathes in a fine spray without having to coordinate their breathing with the release of the drug. This is particularly useful with high-dose inhaled steroids as there is less deposition in the mouth. Nebulisers are sometimes used to treat severe acute attacks of asthma. The use of metered dose inhalers and spacers will be described here.
- Drugs used in the treatment of asthma include bronchodilators, which are used to relieve acute symptoms (for example, salbutamol) and sodium cromoglycate (for example, Intal) and corticosteroids (for example beclomethasone) which are used to prevent attacks occurring.

Normal peak flow readings in adults

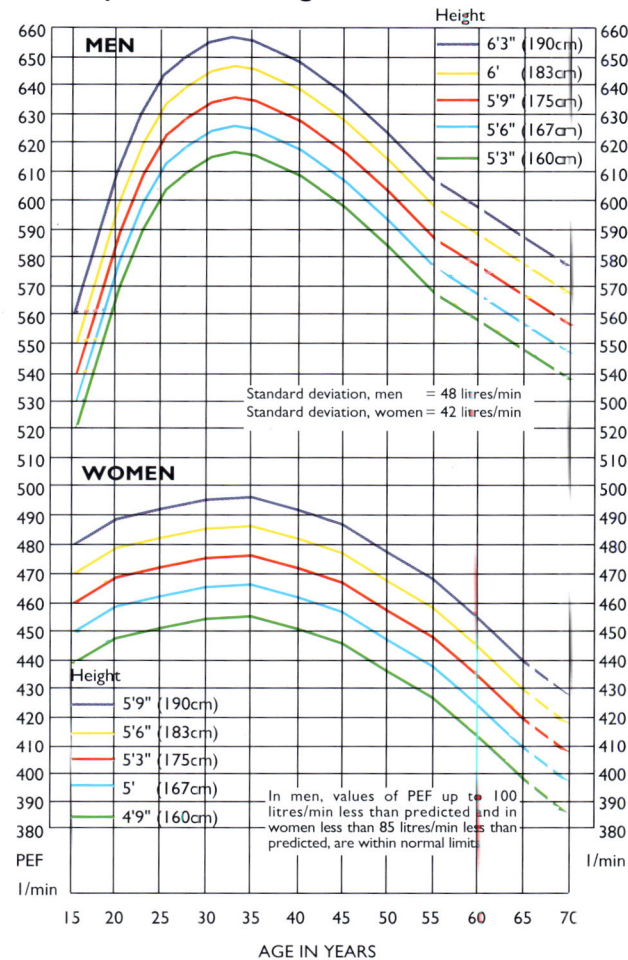

MEN

Height
- 6'3" (190cm)
- 6' (183cm)
- 5'9" (175cm)
- 5'6" (167cm)
- 5'3" (160cm)

Standard deviation, men = 48 litres/min
Standard deviation, women = 42 litres/min

WOMEN

Height
- 5'9" (190cm)
- 5'6" (183cm)
- 5'3" (175cm)
- 5' (167cm)
- 4'9" (160cm)

In men, values of PEF up to 100 litres/min less than predicted and in women less than 85 litres/min less than predicted, are within normal limits

PEF l/min

AGE IN YEARS

Source: Gregg, I., Nunn, A.J. *British Medical Journal* 1973; 3: 3, 282.

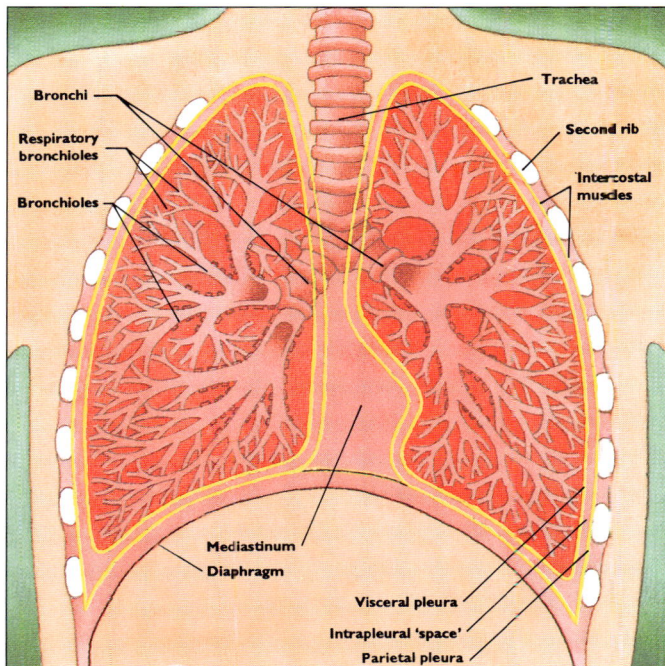

- Bronchi
- Respiratory bronchioles
- Bronchioles
- Trachea
- Second rib
- Intercostal muscles
- Mediastinum
- Diaphragm
- Visceral pleura
- Intrapleural 'space'
- Parietal pleura

USING INHALERS

- The successful use of a metred dose inhaler demands coordination between depressing the canister in the inhaler and breathing in. This can be surprisingly difficult. Try it yourself (with a demonstration inhaler) before attempting to teach the technique.
- Shake the inhaler. Remove the cap over the mouthpiece.
- Breathe out fully but gently.
- With the mouthpiece between the lips, depress the canister at the start of inhalation and continue to breathe in deeply. Hold the breath for 10 seconds.
- Wait 30 seconds before taking a second dose so that the valve in the device returns to normal and will deliver the correct metered dose.
- If the patient is using an inhaled bronchodilator, such as salbutamol, and an inhaled steroid, such as beclomethasone, the bronchodilator should be used first. This is because it relaxes the smooth muscle around the bronchi and allows freer passage of the corticosteroid preventive drugs.

USING A SPACER

- A spacer is especially useful in the treatment of young children and older people with inhaled drugs. The use of a Volumatic will be described here, although there are other similar devices on the market. Always ensure that the device prescribed for the patient is compatible with the size of the inhaler mouthpiece.
- Remove cap and shake inhaler. Insert into the spacer.
- Put the mouthpiece of the Volumatic between the lips. If a child is using the device, gently seal the lips around the mouthpiece by placing your fingers around the lips.
- Depress the canister once to release a dose of the drug.
- As the patient breathes in, a valve allows the drug to pass through the mouthpiece. On expiration the valve closes.
- Hold the breath for about 10 seconds and then breathe in again, but this time without depressing the canister.
- If a child is using the device, a breathing pattern can be established before the canister is depressed. Simply leave the mouthpiece in the child's mouth after the dose has been released until the child has taken several more breaths.

YOU SHOULD NOW FEEL COMPETENT TO

- Measure peak flow rate.
- Teach the use of a metered dose inhaler and a Volumatic.

USEFUL ADDRESSES
Asthma Training Centre, Winton House, Church Street, Stratford-upon-Avon, Warwickshire CV37 6HB.
British Lung Foundation, Kingsmead House, 250 Kings Road, London SW3 5UE.
National Asthma Campaign, 300 Upper Street,, London N1 2XX.

TAKING SMEARS

WHO MAY PRESENT

Any woman to be screened for pre-cancerous changes in the cervix who has been, or is currently, sexually active. (Screening may be offered as part of a formal programme or when a woman presents at the surgery for any other reason.)

PREPARATION

- The woman should be seen in a private room, with a screened-off area for dressing and undressing, where there will be no interruptions.
- She should be asked to empty her bladder beforehand.
- The person taking the smear should assemble the following equipment:
  — Adjustable light
  — Assorted sizes of specula
  — Seamless latex gloves
  — KY jelly
  — Spatulas (Aylesbury are now most used)
  — Frosted end slides
  — Fixative or a pot containing alcohol and 5% acetic acid (deep enough to cover slide)
  — Box for transporting slides
  — Bowl for disposal of specula
  — Request forms
  — Appropriate leaflets
  — Pencil and ballpoint pen (details on the slide should be written in pencil).

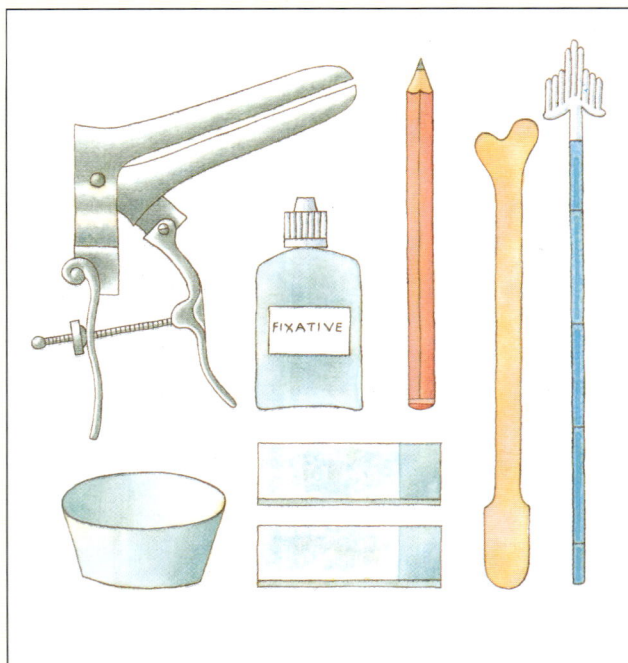

THE INTERVIEW

- Explain the procedure and the reason for it in some detail. This can give the opportunity for the woman to express fears and ask questions.
- Ask for information about general health (for instance, whether the woman smokes, as this increases the risk of cervical cancer).
- Gather information on:
  — Menstrual history
  — Obstetric history
  — Previous smears and gynaecological problems, including any genito-urinary infections
  — Contraceptive history.
- Complete the form accurately. It is vital that any follow-up can be done easily.

TAKIN

- Ensure that the speculum is at body temperature and, if necessary, lubricate it on the sides only with a small amount of lubricant.
- Pass the speculum gently, at the correct angle, rotating through 90° halfway up the vagina, while being aware of the woman's reaction. Do not open the speculum until it is fully inserted. (A very nervous woman may prefer to insert the speculum herself.)
- Visualise the cervix, noting the clinical appearance.
- Rotate the spatula twice through 360°, ensuring that it is well into the os.
- An endocervical brush may be used in conjunction with the spatula but not alone. If both spatula and brush are used, separate slides will be needed.
- Transfer the cells immediately on to a slide and make a good smear — not too thick and not too scanty.
- Flood the slide with fixative and leave for at least five minutes. Alternatively, the slide may be placed immediately in the pot of alcohol with 5% acetic acid.
- Withdraw the speculum gently and offer tissues. Ensure privacy for dressing.

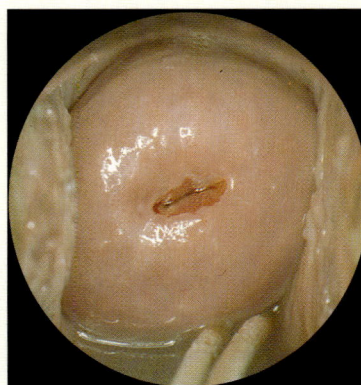

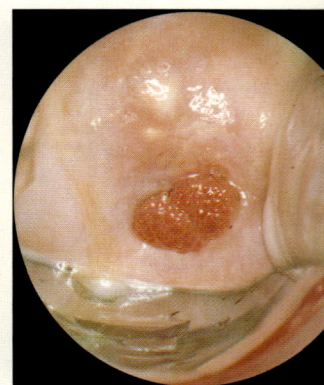

Normal cervix   Tiny polyp in endocervical c

Cancer of the cervix: survival in England and Wales

The five-year relative survival rates for 'all ages' is 58.4

Key:

25–34	
35–44	
55–64	

Source: Cancer Research Campaign. *Factsheet* 9.2. London: CRC, 1988

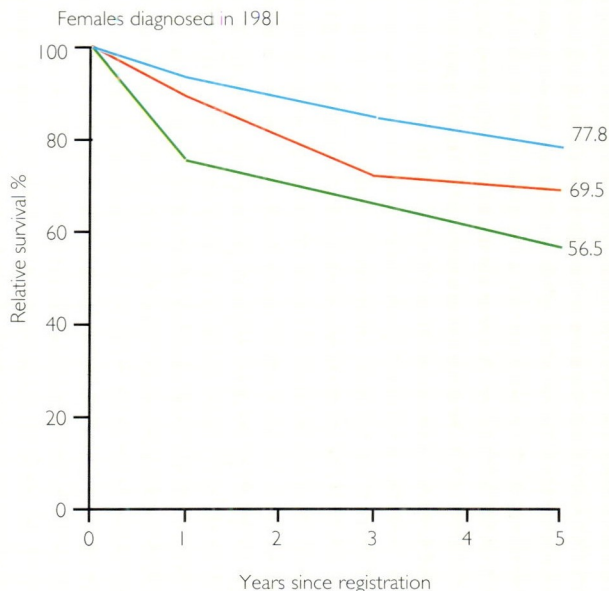

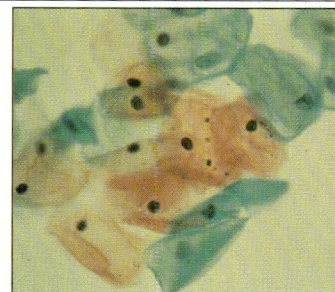

Females diagnosed in 1981

(Graph: y-axis "Relative survival %" from 0 to 100; x-axis "Years since registration" from 0 to 5. End values: 77.8, 69.5, 56.5)

Normal cells

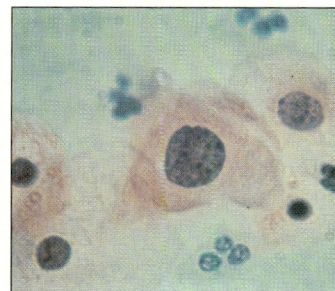

Pre-cancerous cells

WNCCC

SMEAR

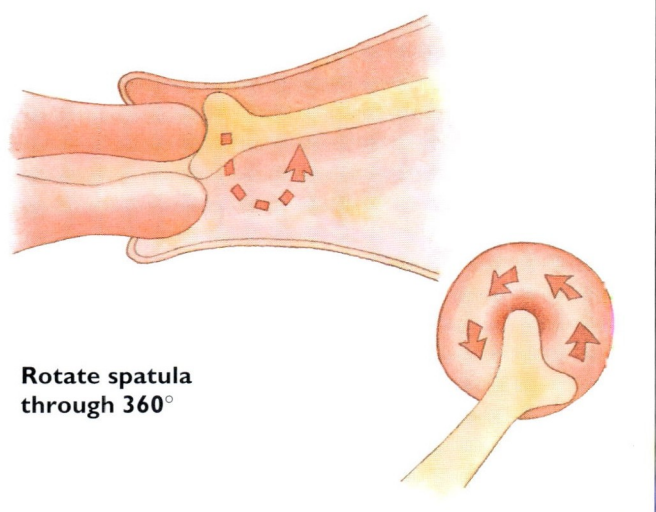

Rotate spatula through 360°

Cervicitis

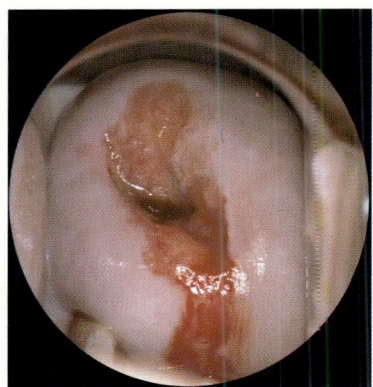

Invasive squamous cancer of cervix

POINTS TO REMEMBER

- Ideally intercourse and use of spermicides should be avoided for 24 hours before the smear is taken.
- Smears are best taken mid-cycle.
- If it is difficult to visualise the cervix, place a folded towel under the woman's buttocks (or get her to place her hands there) in order to tilt the pelvis.
- Smears can also be taken with the woman in the left lateral position.
- A woman with any suspicious lesion on the cervix should be referred to a medical practitioner.
- Any discomfort or pain on intercourse or examination should be referred to the doctor.
- If a woman has not been sexually active, she may not need a smear.
- There is probably a local policy on whether women who have had a hysterectomy should have a vault smear.
- It is recommended that women between the ages of 20 and 64 should have a smear test taken at intervals of between three and five years.

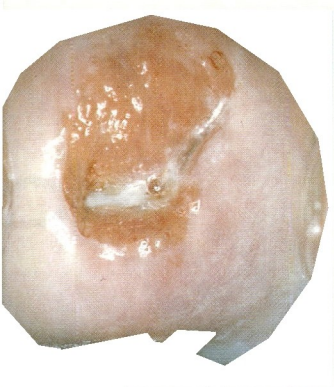

THESE NOTES ARE DESIGNED TO REMIND NURSES OF THE IMPORTANT POINTS TO REMEMBER WHEN TAKING A SMEAR. THEY ARE NOT INTENDED TO BE USED FOR INITIAL TRAINING.

RESOURCES

Cancer Research Campaign. *Fact Sheet*, 13. London: CRC, 1990.
Hopwood, J. *Background to Cervical Cytology Reports* (2nd edition). Burgess Hill: Schering HealthCare, 1991.
Wolfendale, M. *Taking Cervical Smears* (video and booklet £20 or £2 booklet only). Orpington: British Society of Cervical Cytology, 1989.

- Further information about courses can be obtained from the Marie Curie Education Department , 11 Lyndhurst Gardens, London NW3 5NS, to whom acknowledgement is made for help with this article.

PETER GREENHOUSE

COMMON SUMMER AILMENTS

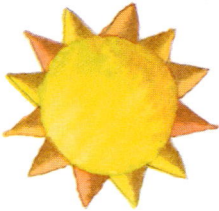

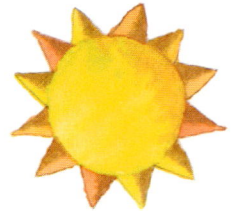

WHO MAY PRESENT?

- Anyone with a minor ailment that has occurred in the summer months
- Any holiday-maker who needs advice on a minor ailment

CONDITIONS THAT OCCUR SEASONALLY

- Some chronic illnesses — for example, chronic obstructive airways disease through increased atmospheric pollution
- Those conditions directly related to the outdoor life, such as heatstroke, sunburn, hives, insect bites, stings and injuries sustained during outdoor activity
- Some infectious diseases which are more common during the spring and early summer — for example, measles, mumps, chicken-pox — although as people gain immunity one is less likely to encounter such diseases
- Diseases contracted abroad, as most people take their main holidays in the summer

ANAPHYLACTIC SHOCK

- Allergic response to insect stings can occur at any time, even in those with no previous history. Systemic reactions can vary from urticaria to severe anaphylactic reaction.
- Symptoms of anaphylactic shock include difficulty in breathing , low blood pressure, tachycardia or arrhythmia, oedema of the face, larynx and tongue and itching skin.
- Adrenaline 1:1000 (to be given by deep intramuscular injection; dosage varies according to age and build) must be available at all times in the treatment room, together with a Brook airway.[1]
- Agree a protocol with the medical staff about the initial assessment and treatment of anyone who may have an anaphylactic reaction — that is, who will do what.

HAY FEVER

Symptoms include rhinitis (runny nose) and conjunctivitis (red, itchy eyes). The onset of hay fever can be between May and August, depending on what sort of grasses and pollens cause the allergy, and symptoms can vary from mild to severe.

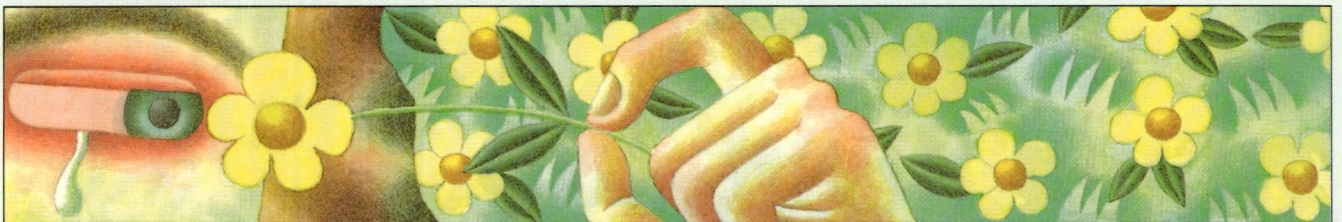

Advise the patient to:
- Stay indoors if possible or avoid the allergen if known
- Wear sunglasses to alleviate eye symptoms
- Take a systemic antihistamine for mild to moderate symptoms. These can be bought over the counter in a pharmacy; the pharmacist can advise on a suitable brand. (If the patient has to pay for prescriptions, buying an over-the-counter brand may be cheaper.) There are now some effective antihistamines which do not cause drowsiness. If it is especially important that the patient is not made drowsy, inhaled steroids may be a more suitable form of treatment
- Use inhaled steroids for more severe nasal symptoms. They will not work for seven to 10 days and must be used regularly, even in the absence of symptoms, to prevent recurrence of the symptoms. This treatment must be medically prescribed
- Use sodium cromoglycate 2% eyedrops for severe allergic conjunctivitis. These have to be used even when the symptoms have abated in order to prevent recurrence. This treatment has to be medically prescribed. The use of ephedrine nasal drops over a long period to relieve nasal congestion is not recommended, as it can lead to a rebound reaction and increased nasal congestion
- Wash the face with cold running water. This washes away the pollen and provides quick relief for itchy eyes and a runny nose.

GASTRO-ENTERITIS

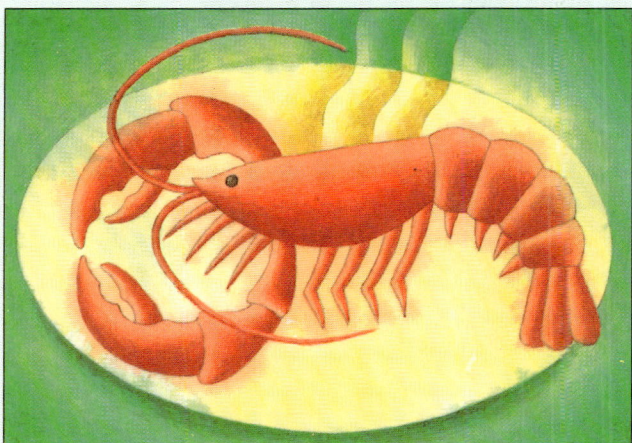

NOTE: THIS SECTION IS NOT CONCERNED WITH THE TREATMENT OF CHILDREN, IN WHOM GASTRO-ENTERITIS CAN QUICKLY LEAD TO DEHYDRATION, WHO WILL NEED CAREFUL ASSESSMENT AND MANAGEMENT.

The number of cases of gastro-enteritis increases in warm weather because bacteria transmitted to food, often by flies, multiplies quickly in warm conditions.

Signs and symptoms include:
- Sudden onset of vomiting, with or without diarrhoea, which can often be related to recently eaten food. (A dietary history is important if more than one member of a family or group is affected. If food is implicated, try to obtain a sample)
- Vomiting, which usually ceases after 24 hours
- Diarrhoea, which may follow the vomiting and in some cases may be the predominant feature of the illness
- Stomach pain.

You should refer to a medical practitioner if:
- The symptoms have persisted longer than 48 hours
- There is a high fever
- There is severe abdominal pain
- There is blood in the stools.

In uncomplicated gastro-enteritis, advise the patient to:
- Eat no solid food for 24 hours
- Drink frequent small amounts of a solution of water, glucose and sodium chloride (which can be bought as a powder, in a sachet, to mix with water)
- After 24 hours gradually introduce solid foods again. (Appetite is a good guide to how much to eat)
- Avoid greasy and spicy foods as well as alcohol
- Pay attention to hygiene measures, such as appropriate hand-washing, and do not prepare foods for the family while the illness persists.

Recovery should be complete in two to three days, although the appetite may not return to normal for several days. If diarrhoea persists, it might be advisable to obtain a stool specimen for culture, so the patient should return if not completely well in a week.

INSECT BITES AND STINGS

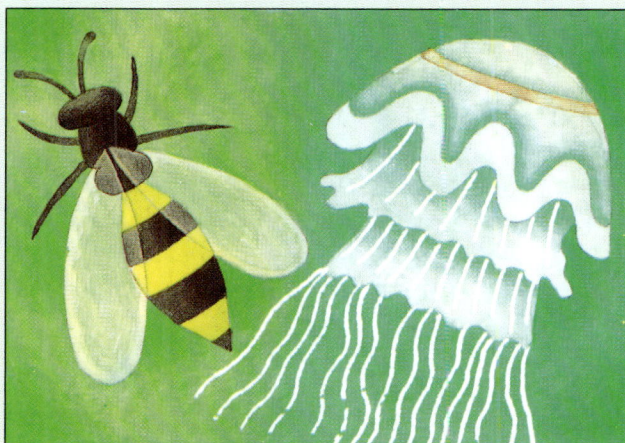

Signs and symptoms:
- A red, raised, itchy area, usually found on the exposed areas of the body. Mosquito or midge bites become more itchy and noticeable after 24–48 hours
- A sting which may be visible in the lump
- Itching which may get worse at night when the skin is warm.

Advice and treatment:
- Whether the wound is infected or not can be difficult to assess because the area will be red and hot anyway. If the surrounding tissue is swollen and red or if you are in doubt, medical advice should be sought.
- Any suggestion of anaphylaxis, especially after a bee sting, requires emergency treatment.
- Be sure to ask if stings and bites were sustained in the UK. There is a risk of malaria even if the correct prophylaxis has been taken.
- Systemic antihistamines are useful in severe but uncomplicated reactions to insect bites. Locally applied antihistamines (creams) are not recommended.
- One per cent hydrocortisone cream (available without prescription) can reduce itching and inflammation.
- In people who are especially susceptible to midge and mosquito bites, it is sensible to cover all exposed areas when out after dark in a warm climate.
- Remember that spiders and ants can bite and that both can cause a severe local reaction.

REMEMBER

If you are in any doubt about your assessment of any of these ailments, get help from a more experienced nurse or from a medical practitioner.

REFERENCE
[1] Department of Health. *Immunisation Against Infectious Disease*. London: HMSO, 1990.

FURTHER READING
Jacobs, M.M., Geels, W. *Signs and Systems in Nursing*. Philadelphia, Pa.: Lippincott, 1985.
Malasanos, L., Barkauskas, C., Stoltenberg-Allen, K. *Health Assessment* (4th edn). St Louis, Mo.: C.V. Mosby, 1990.
Street, S., Burch, K. *Essential Primary Care*. Oxford: Basil Blackwell, 1987.

SCREENING FOR RISKS OF CARDIOVASCULAR DISEASE

WHO MAY PRESENT?

- Any healthy person who wants a check-up
- Someone who is invited by a practice to be screened
- Someone who comes to consult for another reason and whose health awareness can be raised through offering screening

YOU NEED TO KNOW

- The factors that increase the risk of early morbidity and mortality from cardiovascular disease
- How to screen for them
- What to do if you find they are present
- How to explain to the client what you have found
- How to teach the client about self-help measures

RISK FACTORS

It is known that certain factors increase an individual's predisposition to heart disease.

- GENDER
  Men are more likely to develop heart disease at an earlier age
- FAMILY HISTORY
  Having a first-degree male relative who develops heart disease before the age of 50 and a female relative who develops it before the age of 55 increases a person's risk of heart disease
- HIGH BLOOD PRESSURE
  see page 2
- SMOKING
  Carbon dioxide, inhaled from cigarette smoke, causes atherosclerosis
- OBESITY
  Being overweight increases blood pressure and may also be associated with raised lipid levels
- ALCOHOL CONSUMPTION
  High levels of alcohol intake contribute to hypertension
- RAISED LIPID LEVEL
  These might be raised through a diet rich in saturated fats. There may be a family history of the condition hyperlipidaemia which is a metabolic abnormality or the person may have this abnormality without a family history
- SEDENTARY LIFE-STYLE
  Lack of exercise can contribute to obesity and possibly to the effects of stress
- DIABETES
  May predispose to raised cholesterol levels

Alone, each of these factors increases the risk of heart disease. In combination, the risk can increase considerably, as shown in the bar chart.

HOW TO SCREEN FOR RISK FACTORS

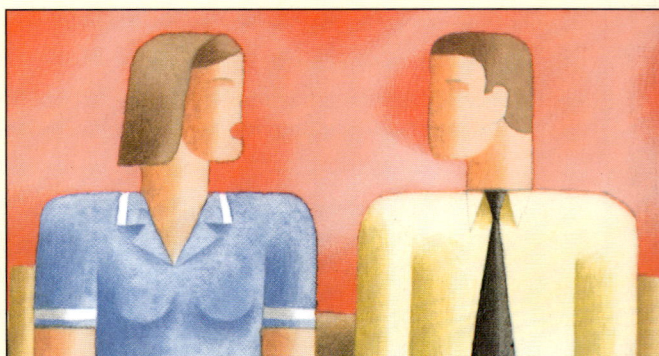

- Discuss relevant factors such as:
  — Smoking: how much, for how long and when the person stopped if an ex-smoker
  — Family history of heart disease
  — Exercise activity
  — Alcohol units consumed per week

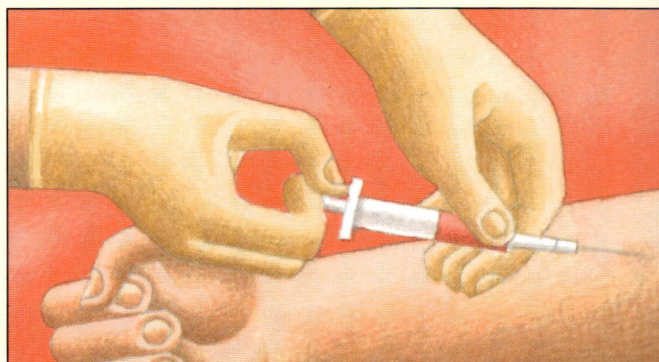

- Measure serum cholesterol in those people who have a high risk of developing heart disease: this will include those with a first-degree relative who had heart disease, those who smoke, those who are overweight and those who are hypertensive

WHAT TO DO IF RISK FACTORS ARE PRESENT

- It will not be helpful to tell someone that his or her risk of heart disease is increased unless that news is accompanied by a plan to decrease the risk
- Remember that blood pressure should be measured three times to get an accurate reading. If the blood pressure is high, treatment should be started by a doctor
- Those who smoke, who are overweight and who take little exercise may be able to change their life-styles and so reduce their risk. It is unlikely to help them if they are made to feel that they are to blame. A better strategy is to explain the risks in terms listeners can understand. Remember to ask whether they have any questions or whether there is anything they do not understand. Be non-judgemental
- Bear in mind that social factors, such as income and peer group pressure, influence life-style behaviours. Try to find out about family life — does a partner smoke, too, for example? Who buys the food? Is the pub a major centre of leisure activity?
- A raised cholesterol level can be lowered by improving the diet in some people. Drugs should be unnecessary except for those with metabolic abnormality

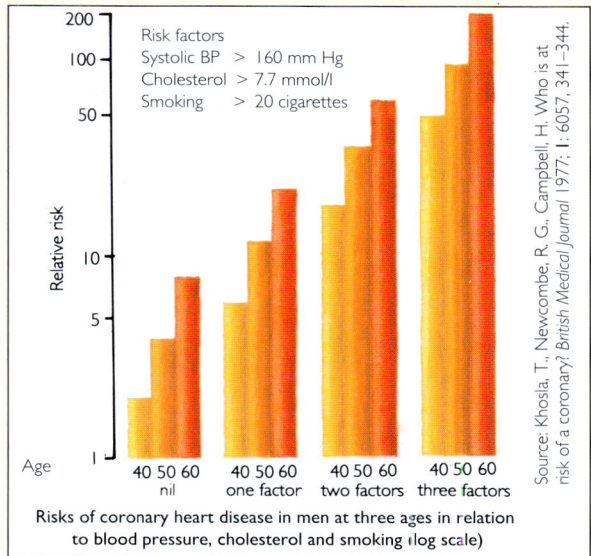

Risk factors
Systolic BP   > 160 mm Hg
Cholesterol   > 7.7 mmol/l
Smoking   > 20 cigarettes

Risks of coronary heart disease in men at three ages in relation to blood pressure, cholesterol and smoking (log scale)

Source: Khosla, T., Newcombe, R. G., Campbell, H. Who is at risk of a coronary? British Medical Journal 1977; I: 6057, 341–344.

- Measure blood pressure accurately. See page 2 to update your knowledge of this

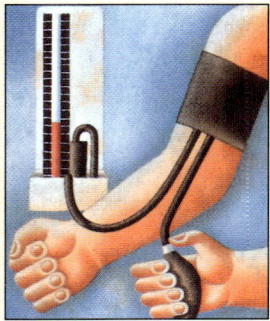

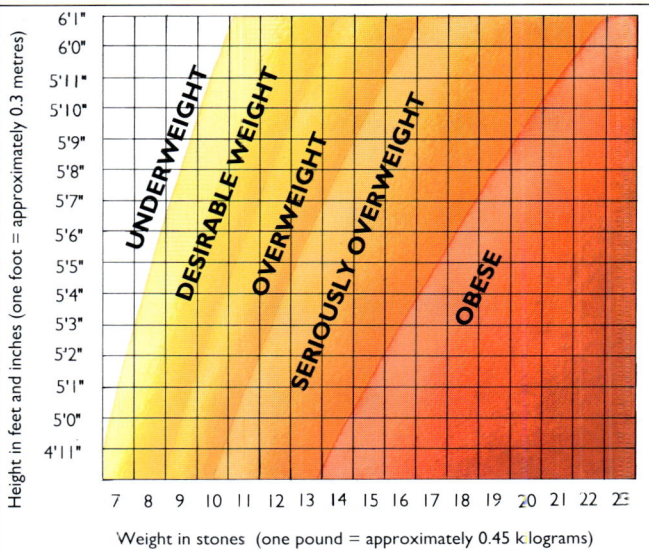

- Check weight. Obesity is most usefully measured by calculating the body mass index (see below). Use accurate scales and metric measurements. To calculate body mass index, divide the weight in kilograms by the height in metres squared:

$$\text{Body mass index} = \frac{\text{Weight in kilograms}}{\text{Height in metres}^2}$$

HELPING ALTER RISK FACTORS

It is clear that, for some people, the only chance of reducing their risk of heart disease lies with them. Here are some hints to help you help your clients.

- Discuss the person's attitude towards his or her life-style
- Give information in a way that is understandable and back it up with literature. A wide range of educational booklets is now available; try your local health promotion department. Be sensitive to the needs of those who have difficulty with reading or understanding English
- Try to find some family support for the person who is changing his or her behaviour. If a partner does the shopping or cooking, see the couple together to discuss diet. If both partners smoke, find out whether they will both try to give up
- Be as well informed as you can be about screening and about risk factors

YOU SHOULD NOW FEEL COMPETENT TO:

- Offer screening for cardiovascular risk factors
- Identify the person who is at high risk of getting cardiovascular disease
- Offer supportive educational measures to those who wish to change their behaviour

FURTHER READING
Coronary Heart Disease: Reducing the Risk. Milton Keynes: Open University, 1987.
Coronary Prevention Group. Risk assessment in the prevention of coronary heart disease. *British Journal of General Practice* 1990; 40 467–469.
Tudor-Hart, J., Stilwell, B., Muir-Gray, I. A. *Prevention of Coronary Heart Disease and Stroke: A Workbook for Primary Care Teams.* London Faber and Faber, 1988.

EAR SYRINGEING

WHO MAY PRESENT?

Anyone who feels deaf and thinks wax may be the cause as:
- They have had wax problems before or someone they know has had a similar problem
- They have been referred by a medical practitioner who has already examined their ears.

TAKING A HISTORY

You need to know:
- Whether the patient has been referred by a doctor
- Whether the patient is self-referred.

Even if the patient has been referred by a doctor, check the history for yourself as:
- The patient may have the instructions confused
- The doctor might have misunderstood what the patient was saying.

Find out:
- Whether there is pain in the ear
- Whether there is deafness
- Whether there is any pain around the ear
- Whether there are any other symptoms, such as giddiness, headache, nausea, itching in the ear or discharge from the ear
- The duration of any symptoms and their severity; for example, does the pain keep the patient awake at night?

Next, you need to know:
- Has the patient had his or her ears syringed before?
- If so, why?
- Has the patient a history of drum perforation?
- If so, when?
- Has the patient a history of otitis externa (infection of the auditory canal)?
- If so, when?

ANATOMY OF THE EAR

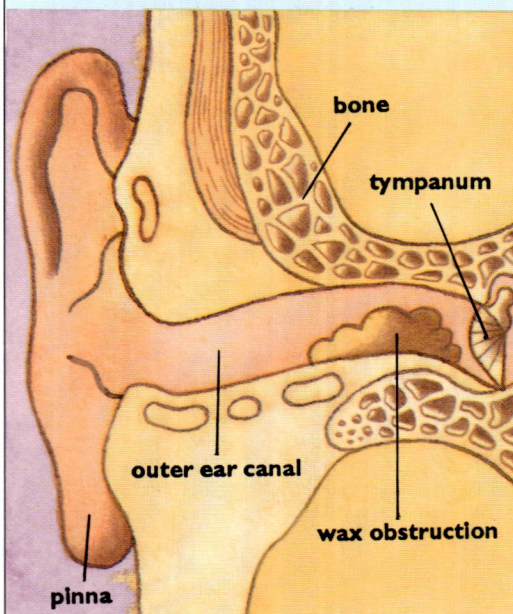

bone

tympanum

outer ear canal

wax obstruction

pinna

HOW TO

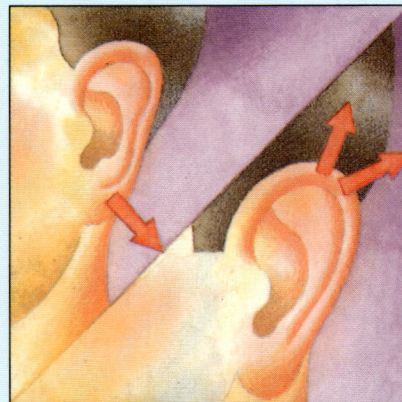

- The patient should be told that the procedure will not be painful but that he or she may experience slight dizziness.
- The patient should be sitting comfortably and covered with something waterproof.
- In the case of a child, pull the pinna down gently to straighten canal.
- In the case of an adult, pull the pinna up and out gently to straighten canal.

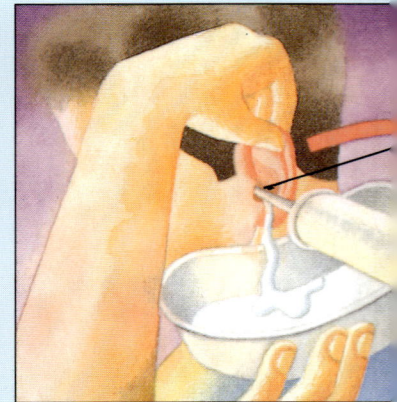

- You should be able to move from [the] chair to the water easily and have unimpeded access to the ear being treated.
- Check that you are using an ear syr[inge] which works — either the tradition[al] sort or an electronic one. Most importantly, the syringe barrel shou[ld] be easy to move and the syringe should not leak.

EXAMINING THE EARS

First, examine the auricle or pinna.
- Inspect the auricle for discharge and any skin lesions.
- Move the auricle up and down and note whether this causes pain.
- Press behind the ear and note whether this causes pain.

Next, examine the ear canal (external auditory meatus) and drum.
- A good auroscope, with a number of different-sized specula, is necessary for this examination.
- Tip the patient's head slightly away from you.
- Use as large an ear speculum as is comfortable for the patient. This will give a better view.
- Gently pull the pinna backwards, upwards and outwards (pulling too hard can be very painful).
- Insert the speculum into the canal, aiming slightly downwards and forwards (too much pressure can be painful).

Identify
- Any wax in the canal — wax can range from sticky and brown to flaky and yellow, with almost any variety in between
- Any foreign body in the canal
- The presence of otitis externa (inflammation of the canal between the eardrum and external opening of the ear which is quite common in swimmers) — the canal will be pale, moist, sometimes swollen and usually tender
- The landmarks of the normal drum, if visible
- Any abnormalities visible.

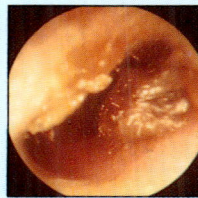

Wax partially occluding drum   Normal drum and canal   Red drum

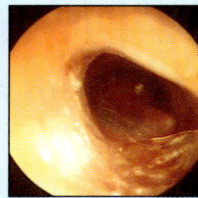

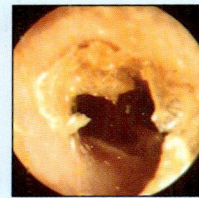

DECIDE WHETHER TO REFER OR SYRINGE

When to refer
- If you suspect otitis media
- If you suspect otitis externa, unless you have a protocol for the identification and treatment of this
- If you identify other symptoms or accompanying deafness when taking the history
- If you see anything unusual in the ear.

When to syringe
- If you have satisfied yourself that there is wax occluding a healthy drum
- If the patient has had this done before and the history and examination reveal no current contraindications
- If the wax is soft enough to be removed easily by syringeing — it may be necessary for the patient to use wax-softening eardrops several times before the procedure takes place.

...GE AN EAR

direct warm water around obstruction

water flow pushes wax out

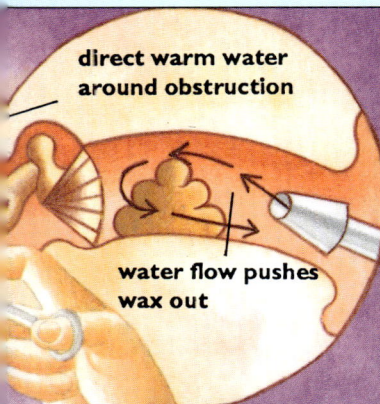

...he syringe should be filled with water ... blood temperature (37°C). The ...ringe should be inserted just into the ...anal, pointing between the canal wall ...nd the obstruction site. The jet of ...ater should be released gently into ...e canal. Too high pressure could ...erforate the drum. Check after each ...ashing. Do not wash for more than ...½–2 minutes.

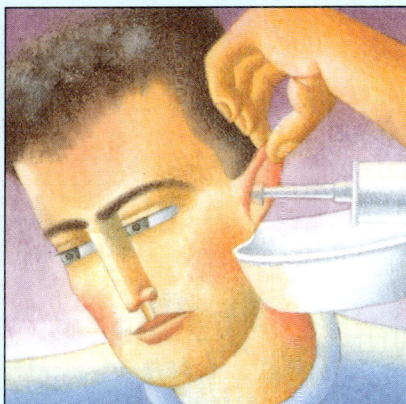

- Collect the water returning from the ear with a suitable bowl, preferably one shaped to fit under the ear. Repeat the procedure until the wax emerges, unless the patient feels pain or discomfort or the wax needs softening.
- Check frequently, using the auroscope, to see whether all the wax has been removed. Ensure that the patient is dry and comfortable afterwards.

NOW YOU SHOULD FEEL COMPETENT TO:

- Understand the indications and contra-indications for ear syringeing
- Take an adequate and appropriate history
- Examine the ear
- Undertake safe and effective ear syringeing
- Refer the patient when necessary.

If you do not feel competent at syringeing ears or you have not done it before, you should ask a nurse or doctor who is experienced in this procedure to watch you perform it. If in doubt as to whom to ask, contact your local community nurse tutors.

FURTHER READING
Bates, B.A. *Guide to Physical Examination and History Taking.* Philadelphia; Lippincott, 1987.

FAMILY PLANNING

WHO MAY PRESENT

- A woman of child-bearing years, a man or a couple who want advice about contraception
- A woman who wants specific information or instruction about a particular method of contraception.

GENERAL POINTS

- Any nurse involved in family planning services must have undertaken a recognised family planning course, such as ENB Course 901.
- Family planning services include not only contraception but also subfertility services and preconceptual counselling. Counselling should also be available as a part of family planning for unplanned pregnancy, abortion, sterilisation, premenstrual syndrome, the menopause and psychosexual needs. These services may have to be made available through referral to suitable agencies.
- Information on contraception should be accurate and unbiased and enable people to enjoy their sexuality. Also the nurse should be sensitive to the possibility of unspoken fears about particular methods.
- This update will deal with two methods of contraception — the contraceptive pill and the condom.

METHODS OF CONTRACEPTION

There are five methods of contraception:
- Hormonal methods, which include combined and progestogen-only oral contraceptives and injectable progestogens
- Barrier methods, such as the condom or the diaphragm
- Mechanical methods, for example, the intra-uterine contraceptive device and withdrawal — when the man ejaculates outside the vagina
- Natural family planning, using the mucous method, the temperature method or the calendar method
- Surgical intervention for male or female sterilisation
- Post-coital contraception, by hormone or by the insertion of an intra-uterine contraceptive device.

Most of these methods of contraception rely on the user to ensure their effectiveness. For example, oral hormonal contraception must be taken correctly and barrier methods used properly if they are to prevent pregnancy. It is therefore vital that instructions are given clearly and are understood.

It is important to remember that contraceptive needs change and depend on the stage of a relationship, the age of the woman, the wish to have children or a certainty that a permanent method of contraception (such as sterilisation) is desirable. Nurses who offer advice and instruction on the use of contraceptive methods should be well informed about their suitability for a range of life situations.

TEACHING ABOUT ORAL CONTRACEPTION

- A woman who has been prescribed an oral contraceptive may consult the nurse for instruction or advice regarding this method of contraception. Ensure that the woman is received into a private environment and have leaflets available in the language which the woman can understand best.
- Check that a full medical history has been taken and an appropriate examination, which should include: checking the blood pressure, weighing the client, examining the breasts and the vagina and taking a cervical smear. Smoking habits should also be noted, as well as the obstetric, gynaecological and menstrual history. Any concurrent medication should be recorded. Check that the client has the contraceptive pill prescribed.
- Ask the client what she knows about the contraceptive pill. Correct any inaccuracies and be sure that she understands the small risks involved in taking the pill. Emphasise that she should report any adverse symptoms to you and the doctor.
- Smoking is known to be associated with an increased risk of circulatory disorders in women taking the combined oral contraceptive pill. It is therefore desirable to offer advice to smokers during a consultation about pill taking. Similarly, obesity is a possible risk factor and, again, appropriate help can be offered.
- Show the pill pack to the client and explain why the days of the week are on it or the pills are of different colours (if the

dose of progestogen is varied, as it is with bi-phasic and tri-phasic pills).
- Explain to the woman when she should take the first pill. With most modern pills, this is usually within 24 hours of the start of menstruation. If this is so, no other contraception is needed from the commencement of the pill. With some older types of pill, it is suggested that the first one is taken on the fifth day of the menstrual cycle, and in this case additional contraceptive methods are needed for the first 14 days. Check the instructions on the pack and, if in any doubt, consult the prescribing doctor.
- Decide with the client what will be a convenient time to take the pill. This is especially important with the progestogen-only pill, when it must be taken at the same time every day to ensure the best contraceptive effect. Shift workers may need particular help with this.
- For women taking a combined oral contraceptive pill, bleeding normally occurs during the pill-free week, although it may be lighter than a period. Use of the progestogen-only pill may result in erratic or absent bleeding. These variations should be discussed.
- Explain the possible side-effects of hormonal contraception, such as sore breasts, nausea, spotting or headaches, and reassure the woman that these should diminish with each cycle. Explain that a change is possible if symptoms persist.

ORAL HORMONAL CONTRACEPTION

- There are two types of oral hormonal contraception: combined oestrogen–progestogen pills and progestogen-only oral ones.
- The mode of action of the combined pill is primarily to suppress ovulation by inhibiting the secretion of follicle-stimulating hormone and luteinising hormone. There is no longer a true menstrual cycle. Instead, bleeding occurs during the pill-free days because of hormone withdrawal. The combined pill has other contraceptive effects: it changes the endometrium, which prevents implantation of a fertilised ovum; alters the normal motility of the Fallopian tubes; and inhibits the progression of sperm through the cervical mucous.
- Progestogen-only pills act mainly by making the cervical mucous hostile to sperm and by changing the endometrium, so that implantation of a fertilised ovum cannot occur.

MISSED PILLS

- **Combined oral contraceptives.** If a pill is taken more than 12 hours late, other precautions should be used for the following seven days. In addition, if pills are missed during the last seven days of active pills, the next pack should be started without a break.
- **Progestogen-only pills.** If a pill is taken two to three hours late, other precautions should be taken for 48 hours.
- If vomiting occurs within three hours of taking the pill, or there is persistent diarrhoea, additional contraceptive precautions should be taken as advised above. (Note that if a woman is able to retain another combined oral contraceptive pill within 12 hours, the level of contraceptive effectiveness will not be affected. The time limit for progestogen-only pills is three hours.)
- If other medication is prescribed at any time, the woman should take her pills to the surgery or pharmacy to check whether there is likely to be an interaction which could reduce effectiveness. She should be aware that additional contraceptive precautions may be needed.

THE CONDOM

- The use of a condom should preferably be explained to both partners.
- A condom pack should show a British Standards Kite Mark and a date of expiry.
- Condoms are reliable if used throughout the menstrual cycle and if put on correctly.
- They may protect against cervical cancer and give protection against sexually transmitted diseases, including AIDS.
- To use a condom correctly:
  — It should be removed carefully from the packet, ensuring that the condom does not tear.
  — It should be put on before there is any vaginal or vulval contact.
  — For maximum effectiveness a spermicidal cream should be used (by the woman). The cream must be water-based, as oil-based creams will damage the rubber.
  — The condom should be unrolled on to the erect penis, with the closed end held between finger and thumb to expel the air. Care should be taken not to tear the condom with fingernails, rings or rough skin on the hands.
  — After intercourse, the penis should be removed from the vagina while it is still slightly erect, so that the condom is still in place. The condom should be held firmly at the base.
  — The condom should be removed well clear of the woman's vulva so that accidental spillage of semen cannot occur.
- Advise clients that, if the condom tears during intercourse, post-coital contraception should be sought.

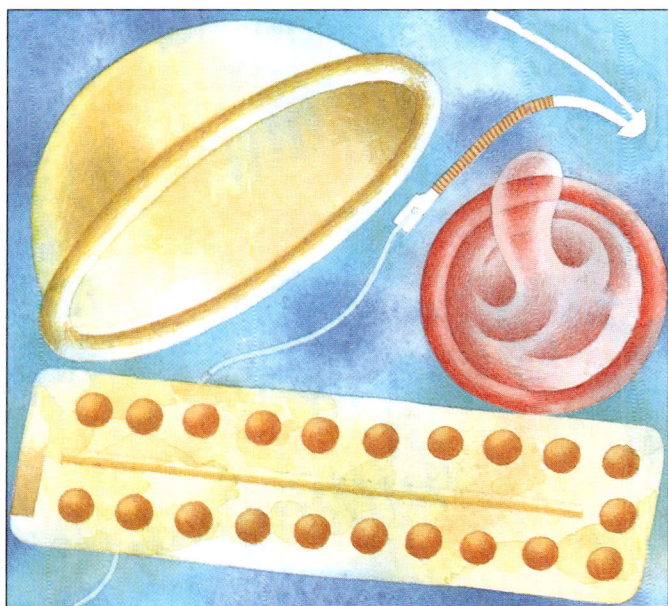

NOW YOU SHOULD FEEL COMPETENT TO:

- Give clients accurate information about the contraceptive pill and the condom.
- Instruct clients in the safe use of the condom as a method of contraception.

FURTHER READING
Carne, S., Day, K., Elstein, M. et al. Handbook of Contraceptive Practice. Heywood: Department of Health, 1990.
Kilby, D. Manual of Safe Sex, Philadelphia, Pensylvania.: B.C. Decker Inc., 1986.
RCN Family Planning Forum. Family Planning Manual for Nurses, Harrow: Scutari, 1991.
RCN Family Planning Forum. Family Planning Nursing. Harrow: Scutari, 1989.
Roberts, A. Systems of Life: reproductive system. Nursing Times 1991; **87**: 41, 45–48.